Easy Eating: A Clear Guide to Nutrition, Healthy Food, Wellness and Balanced Diet for a Fit Heart and a Strong Body

Simple Strategies for a Heart-Healthy Diet and Making Smart Food Choices

Glenda K. Ashworth

ISBN: 9798379037307

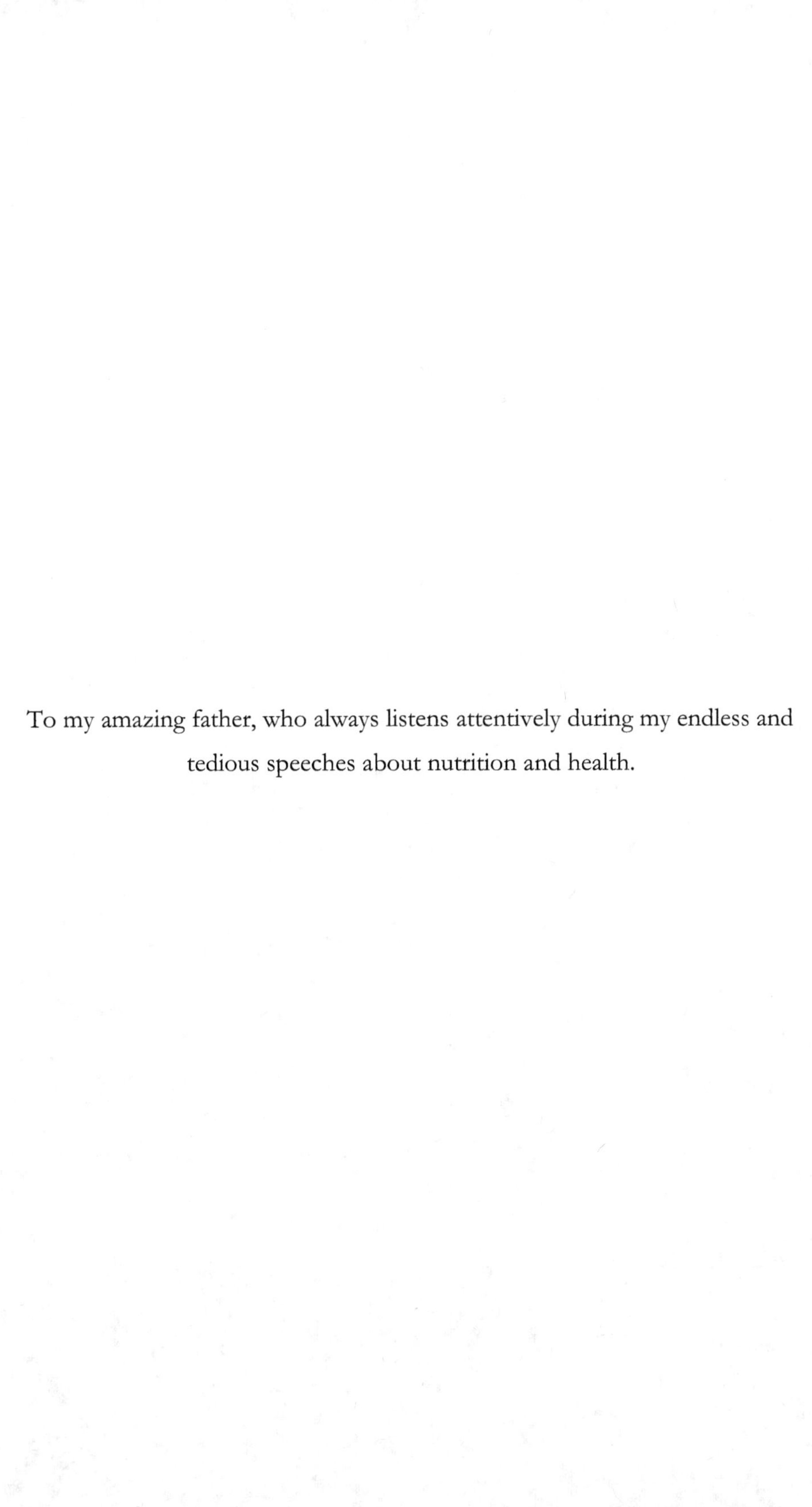

To my amazing father, who always listens attentively during my endless and tedious speeches about nutrition and health.

CONTENTS

Acknowledgments

I would also like to extend my heartfelt appreciation to my colleagues at work, who have helped me in the creative process by contributing their ideas and suggestions, which are ultimately reflected in this publication.

Last, I would like to thank my family for their patience in reading and re-reading the pages of this book, providing me with their valuable feedback to make it more understandable to all readers.

1

INTRODUCTION

Eating healthy is not as difficult as we have been led to believe. At least, it is not so much if we educate ourselves on simple concepts and principles that can help us make healthy decisions about the foods we eat. Throughout this book, we will see and develop several of these ideas, but first, I would like to begin by explaining, with a simple premise, how we can identify healthy food. Generally, foods are healthier the less they are altered from their natural state. The more natural a food is, the fewer ingredients it has (or none at all). Let's look at some practical examples:

- A fresh apple is healthier than apple juice with added sugar.
- A grilled chicken breast is healthier than a breaded nugget fried in refined flour and seed oil.
- A raw peanut is healthier than industrial peanut butter.

So, while it is important to pay attention to the ingredients list and the nutrients in a food product, it is not the most important thing.

The most important thing is to understand that raw materials and unprocessed or minimally processed foods are usually healthier than their ultra-processed alternatives.

We may also come across processed (but not ultra-processed) healthy products, such as natural yogurt, canned legumes, hummus, or even extra-virgin olive oil. Yes, these products have undergone some processing to become what they are: they have been fermented, crushed or decanted, or an acidic or salty solution has been added to prevent the proliferation of microorganisms. This does not mean they are unhealthy, far from it.

However, the same cannot be said for ultra-processed products, which are usually made with a very long list of ingredients: flours (whether wheat, oats, spelt, rye), fats or oils (olive, sunflower, palm), sugar (with many synonyms we will learn about later), salt, additives (preservatives, colorants, sweeteners, gasifiers).

Now that we've cleared that up, let's talk about non-communicable diseases to understand better one of the main topics we will cover in this book. Non-communicable diseases are those that do not spread from person to person and are responsible for most deaths in Western countries. Many of these diseases are preventable, are related to lifestyle, and modifiable risk factors, such as lack of physical activity, poor diet, smoking, excessive alcohol consumption and stress. Among the most common and preventable non-communicable diseases are type 2 diabetes, chronic obstructive pulmonary disease (COPD), chronic kidney disease, cancer, and cardiovascular diseases (CVD).

It may sound like bad news, right? Well, it is bad news. These diseases have been on the rise in recent years and cause a lot of pain and suffering. But not everything is bad news, as they can mostly be prevented by adopting healthy habits that are usually the same for all pathologies. Exercising is good not only for preventing type 2 diabetes but also for overall health. Similarly, quitting smoking is not only good for the lungs but also great for the body. Likewise, healthy eating will not only decrease our chances of having a heart attack but also make it less likely for us to develop any of these non-communicable diseases.

Of all these diseases, cardiovascular diseases, which include heart and circulatory system diseases, are the leading cause of death worldwide. That's why, throughout these pages, we will focus primarily on nutrition regarding these pathologies, although we will also talk about health in general.

Cardiovascular Diseases

If there is one thing to remember regarding cardiovascular diseases (CVD), it is that they are multifactorial. We will need multidisciplinary strategies to prevent or combat them. So, although this document aims to determine what dietary guidelines could help reduce cardiovascular risk (CVR), it would be of little use to focus only on this aspect if we overlook other equally significant factors and do not focus on what really matters: lifestyle habits. A good diet is not very useful if one smokes, drinks alcohol and is sedentary.

Traditionally, dietary guidelines aimed at reducing cardiovascular risk focused on reducing fat or lipid intake, and more specifically, saturated fat and cholesterol intake. This demonization of fats was largely due to the Seven Countries Study carried out in the 1970s. This and other studies of that time laid the groundwork for the epidemiology of CVD. So much so that even today, the dietary recommendations of many healthcare professionals are still based on them. However, in the more than 50 years since then, knowledge about the pathophysiology of CVD has increased significantly, and these guidelines, once useful, have become outdated.

It is common to find healthcare professionals who, when faced with patients with a history of CVD, implement dietary guidelines such as eliminating nut intake because they are too fatty, removing eggs because they are high in cholesterol, recommending skimmed dairy products because they are low in fat, or prescribing a glass of wine a day because it is cardioprotective. Historically, research on cardiovascular risk factors has been fraught with confounding factors not taken into account because this research has focused on specific nutrients such as saturated fats. But people do not eat nutrients; they eat foods that, ultimately, are matrices that have an enormous amount of substances, among which there are nutrients, yes, but also various types of xenobiotic substances that can play a fundamental role in our health (tannins, insoluble fiber, flavonoids, etc.). The population does not eat proteins and fats with carbohydrates for breakfast; they eat milk with cereals.

The recommendations to be given should focus on foods and not on the macronutrients they have. Making nutrient recommendations to the general population is not only very reductionist but counterproductive. People do not know what a monounsaturated fat is or what starch or eicosapentaenoic acid (EPA) are, but they know what olive oil, potatoes or salmon are. However, olive oil is not just oleic acid, potato is not just starch, and salmon is not just omega-3. They are complex matrices that have a multitude of substances of various natures that can interact with the body in various ways. Still, it is advisable to know the main nutrients that can have implications for cardiovascular health.

Although we will learn basic notions about the nutrients that make up the food we put in our mouths, we will focus on the foods themselves and learn to distinguish between those that are healthy and those that are not.

2

NUTRIENTS INVOLVED IN HEALTH

Fiber

Fiber plays a role in fat metabolism by decreasing serum cholesterol levels and the fraction bound to LDL (the so-called "bad cholesterol"). This is due to changes in the speed of intestinal transit caused by fiber consumption, the creation of short-chain fatty acids by the microbiota (the famous gut flora), and plant sterols in foods that have fiber, among other causes. For every 5-10 g of soluble fiber, LDL cholesterol concentrations decrease by 5-10%. So logical recommendations would be aimed at promoting the consumption of minimally processed plant-based products (fruits, vegetables, legumes, whole grains and nuts). A high intake of simple sugars is associated with a decrease in HDL cholesterol ("good cholesterol") and an increase in VLDL (another "bad cholesterol") and triglycerides, which are not recommended in diets to reduce cardiovascular risk.

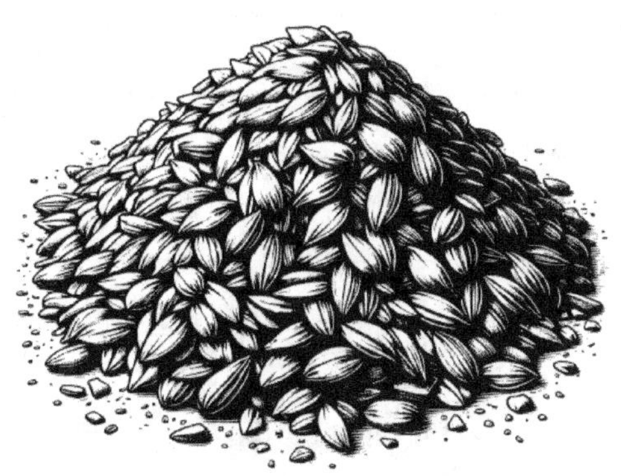

The same happens with foods rich in complete carbohydrates devoid of fiber (refined flours), which are digested, breaking down into simple sugars quickly and producing a peak in blood sugar levels (increase in blood sugar) with a consequent elevation of insulin. Dietary strategies should be aimed at replacing refined flour-rich foods and ultra-processed products with whole grains, fruits, nuts, legumes and vegetables.

Saturated Fats

Saturated fats have been enemy number one of CVD from the outset. However, this viewpoint is very simplistic. Dairy products have a lot of saturated fat; do they promote the development of CVD? Apparently not. How is this possible? Firstly, we must contextualize and determine which dairy product we are talking about. Eating plain yogurt is not the same thing as eating a custard. Similarly, it is not the same thing to drink a glass of whole milk as a sugary milkshake. Differences? Some are lightly processed foods, while others have added sugar. This factor is not considered when dietary recommendations on dairy products are given. It is not useful to tell the patient to consume a dairy serving per day if the dairy products they consume are full of sugar.

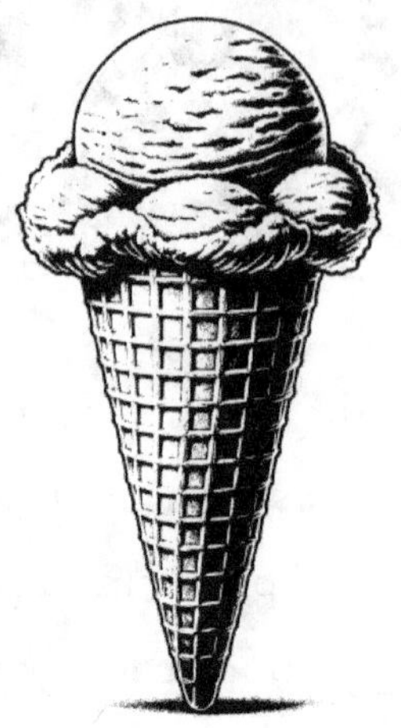

Secondly, it is worth knowing that the fatty acids that have been related to atherogenic and thrombogenic potential (to understand, those that favor the appearance of clots and atheroma plaques) are long-chain saturated fatty acids (from most to least atherogenic: myristic, palmitic, and lauric, while stearic acid could be considered neutral). However, medium and short-chain fatty acids do not seem to influence this aspect. What foods (or food products) are rich in long-chain fatty acids? Pastry products, ice cream, desserts... Does this mean that a doughnut is bad for cardiovascular health because it has saturated fat? No, because the doughnut not only has long-chain saturated fats, it also has free sugar, refined flour, and trans fats... I emphasize the doughnut to make it clear that food is much more than an isolated nutrient or group of nutrients, as mentioned in the introduction.

Returning to dairy products, don't they have long-chain saturated fats and not favor CVD? Yes, they contain this type of fat. However, they are not related to CVD, and, for example, in the case of fermented dairy products such as kefir or natural yogurt, they even seem to prevent them to some extent. This may be because dairy products also have monounsaturated and polyunsaturated fatty acids, as well as other bioactive compounds found in their lipid fraction. And in the case of fermented dairy products, it may be due to the fermentation process itself and the resulting substances. But it is not known for certain what makes whole dairy products neutral and fermented dairy products protective.

This same pattern is repeated on countless occasions in epidemiology and nutrition. For example, fruits are healthy because of their high content of antioxidant substances; however, if antioxidant substances are taken as supplements, mortality increases (sounds paradoxical, doesn't it?).

For all these reasons, I repeat the idea that food is much more than a nutrient or a set of them, hence the difficulty of accurately determining what makes a food healthy or not.

Monounsaturated Fats

The quintessential monounsaturated fat is oleic acid. Sources of this fatty acid include avocados, nuts and virgin olive oil. Contrary to popular belief, oleic acid does not have a significant effect on plasma lipids, at least from a strictly purist perspective. However, consuming virgin olive oil is associated with a decreased risk of cardiovascular disease. This could be due to the antioxidants it contains, such as polyphenols.

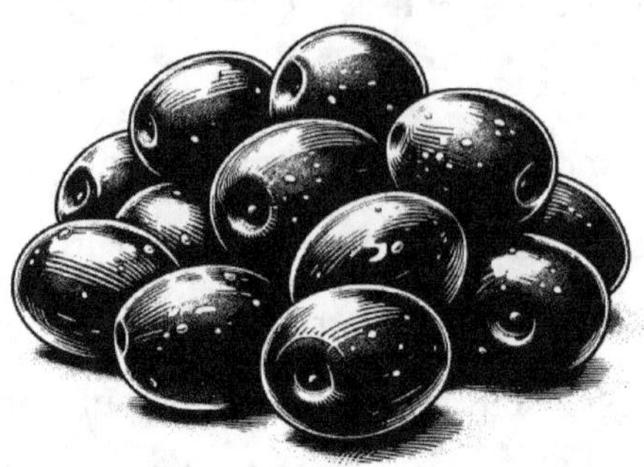

In addition, it is the oil of choice for cooking due to its high resistance to high temperatures. Virgin olive oil is also associated with antithrombotic effects (reduced platelet aggregation, increased fibrinolysis, etc.) and improved insulin sensitivity. Another source of oleic acid is ham; however, ham is not just oleic acid: it is a processed meat with a high salt content and an overall unfavorable lipid profile.

Polyunsaturated Fats

Among these fats, we can highlight omega-3 and omega-6 fatty acids. The most common omega-6 fatty acid is linoleic acid, which is present in seed oils (like sunflower oil or corn oil, for example). The omega-3 fatty acid α-linolenic acid is abundant in nuts (especially walnuts) and in oils such as soybean, canola and flaxseed. Both fatty acids are essential, meaning we need to incorporate them into our body through our diet. However, excess linoleic acid (omega-6) is associated with pro-inflammatory effects, while α-linolenic acid (omega-3) is associated with lower rates of coronary heart disease and decreased mortality.

But we have omega-3 fatty acids from fish oil or fat, which are eicosapentaenoic acid (EPA) and docosahexaenoic acid (DHA). They are associated with anti-inflammatory, antithrombotic, and anti-chemotactic effects and are not essential as they are synthesized from α-linolenic acid mentioned earlier. Additionally, they are associated with decreased plasma triglycerides.

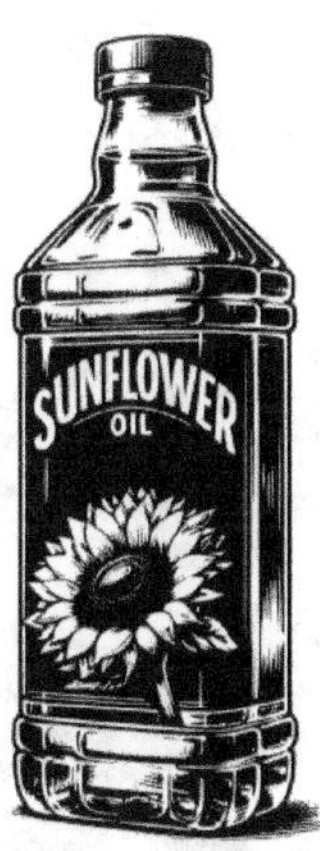

One special mention deserves the high oleic sunflower oil. Unlike its "sibling" the common sunflower oil, high oleic sunflower oil is rich in oleic acid (it was obvious, right?), which, as we have seen, is a monounsaturated fat, like in olive oil. This makes this oil less unhealthy than common sunflower oil and favors its resistance to high temperatures, so it's used to fry food safely. But, what happens with most seed oils is that, when used for frying, they generate toxic products, such as aldehydes and polar compounds, whose regular consumption can be harmful to health.

Trans Fats

Trans fats can be found naturally in meats and dairy products. In these cases, they are not strongly associated with CVD, especially when consumed in moderation. However, trans fats found in ultra-processed products (predominantly elaidic acid) such as baked goods, cookies, processed foods, breakfast cereals, sliced bread and hamburgers are associated with decreased HDL cholesterol and increased levels of CRP, interleukin-6, LDL cholesterol, triglycerides, and lipoprotein A (meaning they are not recommended).

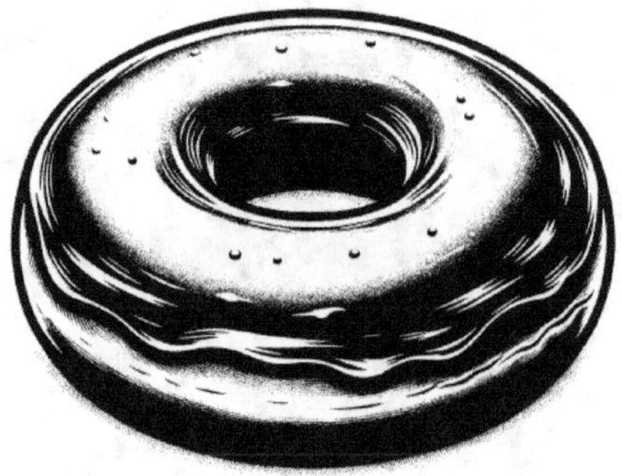

It is advisable to avoid all types of ultra-processed foods in general, but if we focus on trans fatty acids, the ultra-processed products with the highest amounts of trans fats are usually industrial popcorn, margarine and donuts.

Cholesterol

Cholesterol has been one of the most demonized substances in terms of dietary recommendations given in recent years. This has led to commonly held beliefs, such as the idea that eggs are one of the worst foods for patients with cardiovascular disease. It is known that dietary cholesterol causes a moderate increase in blood cholesterol, unlike what happens with trans fats or long-chain saturated fatty acids.

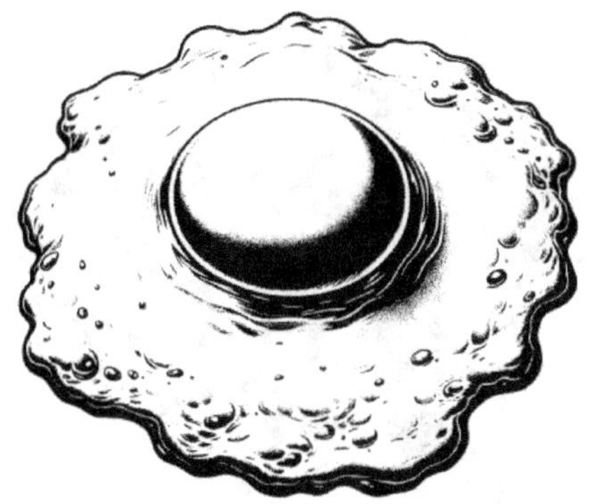

However, there is still no clear relationship between dietary cholesterol intake and cardiovascular risk. Various studies have shown that egg consumption seems to be neutral not being associated with an increased risk of cardiovascular disease. Although eggs are high in cholesterol, a lipid profile makes them less atherogenic. Paradoxically, when considering cardiovascular health, it is preferable to have scrambled eggs for breakfast instead of sugary cereals and cookies.

Plant Sterols or Stanols

Plant sterols or stanols have a low intestinal absorption rate. However, due to their structural similarity to cholesterol, they compete with cholesterol at the intestinal level, displacing it from micelles and reducing its absorption by around 30%. They are also related, for this same reason, to a reduction in LDL cholesterol (remember, "bad cholesterol"). They are present in legumes, fruits, nuts, vegetables and oils.

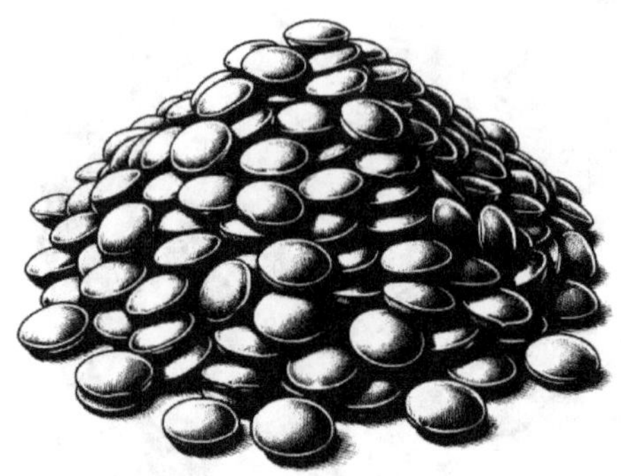

3

FOODS TO AVOID

All right, now we're more informed and aware of some nutrients that play a role in our health, which can come in handy when enhancing a dinner with friends. However, the recommendations in this book aimed at achieving a fit heart and a strong body won't focus on these nutrients because humans don't eat nutrients; we eat food. So let's now examine the foods we should avoid in our daily lives.

Ultra-Processed Foods

Ultra-processed products are characterized by being highly palatable foods made with many ingredients, where refined flours, low-quality fats, salt, and sugar predominate. They occupy a large percentage of supermarket shelves and are a public health problem, as they are associated with overweight and obesity, hypertension, type 2 diabetes mellitus, and inflammation and metabolic syndrome. Examples of ultra-processed foods include pizzas, pastries, hamburgers, cold cuts or cured meats, most spreadable cheeses, sausages, sandwich bread, burger or hot dog buns, breakfast cereals, cookies and so on.

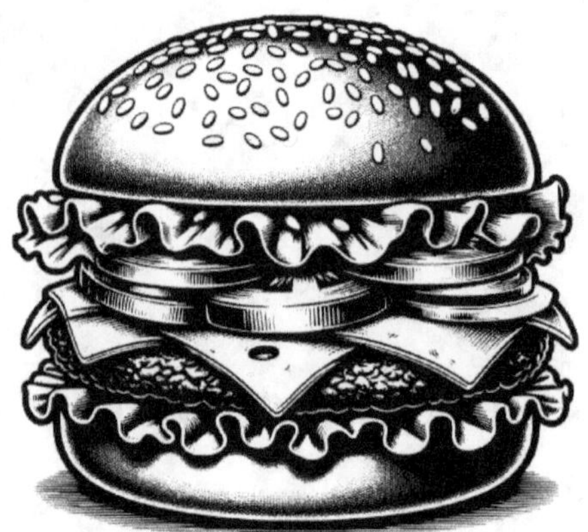

Since we are talking about ultra-processed products, we cannot avoid talking about the famous palm oil. We have all heard of this oil and its bad reputation (and for good reason). Usually, if we see it in the ingredients, we should not buy the product, not only because refined palm oil (which reaches our supermarkets) is bad for our health but also because palm oil is generally present in the ultra-processed products, especially in pastries and biscuits, which are generally unhealthy even if they have palm oil or not. Palm oil usually appears in ingredients under this same name or similar ones, such as vegetable fat (palm), palm fat, palm kernel, palm stearin, and palm butter.

Salt

Limiting salt intake is essential in patients with cardiovascular disease. However, most of the salt consumed by the population comes not from the saltshaker but from ultra-processed foods (processed meat, snacks, bread, cheese, and prepared meals, mainly). The goal, then, is not so much to reduce salt from the saltshaker but to reduce the consumption of "hidden" salt.

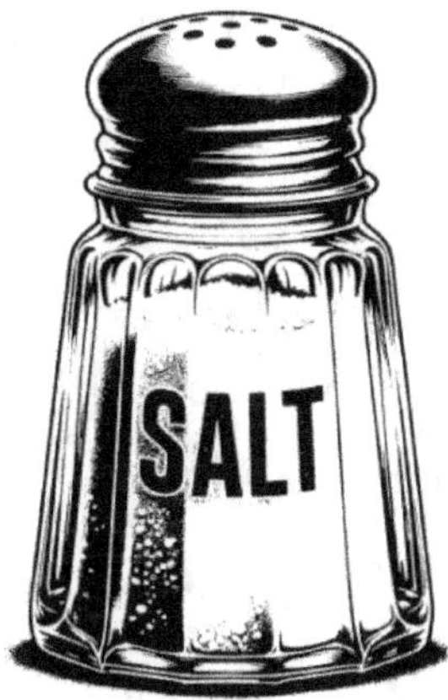

How do we know if a food has a high amount of salt? Well, to find out, it's essential that in addition to looking at the ingredient list, we go to the nutrition information table and check the grams of salt it has. We can group food products into three categories based on the amount of salt they have:

- High salt: 1.25 g or more.
- Moderate salt: between 0.25 and 1.25 g.
- Low salt: 0.25 g or less.

If a proper diet aimed at reducing cardiovascular risk is followed, adding a pinch of salt to certain dishes does not seem worrisome (focusing on iodized salt over common salt, unless contraindicated). However, replacing salt with spices such as turmeric, garlic powder, curry, onion powder, rosemary, or thyme can also be useful.

Sugar

The WHO recommends limiting sugar intake to no more than 25 grams per day. This means that the less sugar consumed, the better. We are talking about a limit, not a minimum recommendation for consumption. Sugar is unnecessary for the brain. What the brain needs is glucose, which it obtains easily from all the foods we consume. When we talk about these WHO recommendations for limiting sugar consumption, we are referring to free sugar found in ultra-processed foods, "soft drinks," "energy drinks," pastries, cookies, sweetened dairy products, or breakfast cereals. The intrinsic sugar in fruit, naturally present in it, would not fall into this classification.

And the truth is that fruit is healthy, not related to overweight or obesity and we shouldn't worry about its intrinsic sugar (we are referring to natural and whole fruit we need to chew, not juices, jams, or preserves). Generally, the industry knows that we are trying to reduce our sugar consumption more and more. So euphemisms or synonyms of sugar or similar compounds are sometimes used.

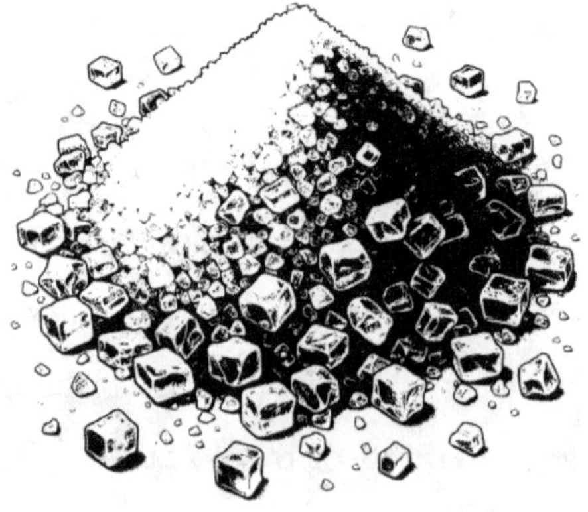

To detect hidden sugars in a food product, we should be suspicious when we read:

- It has syrups (such as fructose, corn, glucose, sap, agave, maple, etc.).
- That there are monosaccharides or disaccharides, such as fructose, glucose, maltose, isomaltose, dextrose (notice that all end in -ose).
- Words such as molasses, cane crystals, dextrins, or maltodextrins.

Processed Meat

Consumption of these products should be avoided. They have a high salt content, unhealthy fats (as well as other substances) and are related to increased cardiovascular risk. In addition, their consumption promotes the development of colorectal cancer. We are referring to sausages, cold cuts, and deli meats.

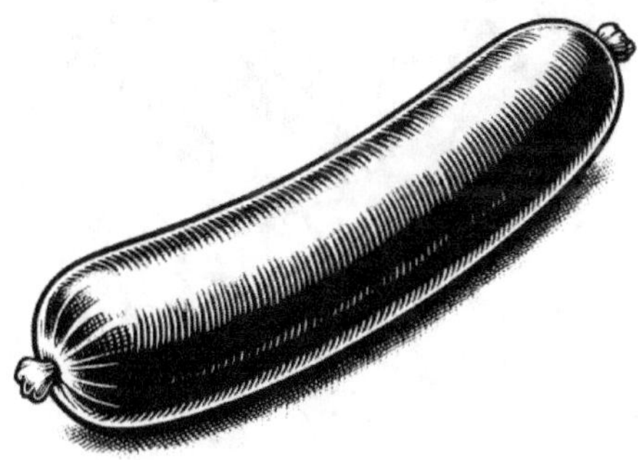

Red Meat

In the same way, as with cold cuts and processed meats, the consumption of red meat is also associated with cardiovascular risk and colorectal cancer. However, this association is not as strong or, at least for now, does not have as much scientific evidence. That's why we talk about avoiding processed meats and moderating the consumption of red meat.

Moderate consumption of red meat could be one or two servings per month, at most, of about 120 grams net weight. As with sugar, we are talking about a maximum not to be exceeded. The less red meat we consume, the better. Beef, veal, lamb, or pork are examples of red meats.

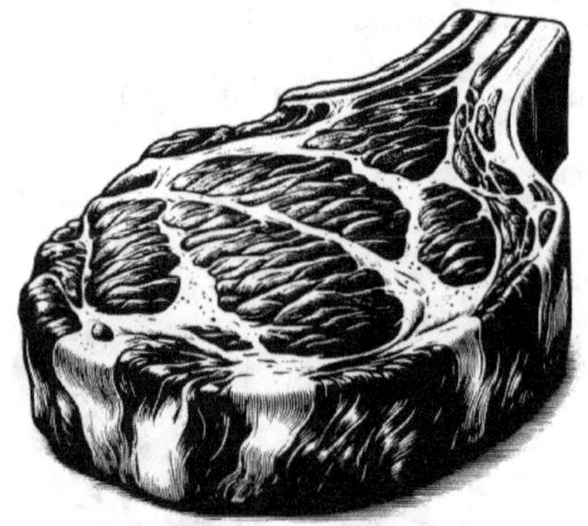

Alcohol

Unlike what has been said in recent years, alcohol is not cardioprotective in any dose. It is not the same for our health to have a glass of wine as to have three glasses of rum, but this does not mean that wine is healthy. One glass of wine a day could be compatible with a good diet, but promoting its consumption is not responsible since alcohol is not only not cardioprotective, but it is also a neurotoxic and carcinogenic substance. If we want a patient to consume tannins (the compound to which these false cardioprotective properties of wine were attributed), why not recommend that they consume red grapes instead of wine? That wine has tannins does not neutralize the 12 or 14% alcohol it has.

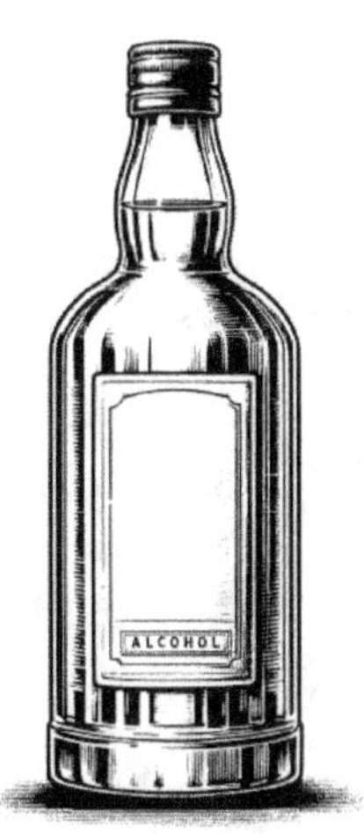

4

RECOMMENDED FOODS

Nuts

Nuts (such as walnuts, cashews, hazelnuts, pistachios, etc.) reduce the risk of cardiovascular diseases. They boast an excellent composition of fatty acids and have significant fiber, antioxidant vitamins (like vitamin E), magnesium, folic acid, arginine, and calcium, among others. They have antiplatelet properties (preventing blood clot formation) and lipid-lowering effects (reducing bad fats in the blood)and antiarrhythmic actions (helping to regulate heart rhythm), and improving endothelial function (enhancing the health of the inner layer of blood vessels, essential for proper blood circulation). Consuming nuts is also associated with a lower risk of cancer, respiratory diseases, diabetes, and infections. It's best to consume them raw or roasted and avoid eating them fried, salted, or caramelized.

Did you know something curious? Despite their high content of good fats, nut consumption is not associated with overweight or obesity, partly due to their satiating effect and high fiber content, making them suitable for weight loss diets (even if it seems paradoxical).

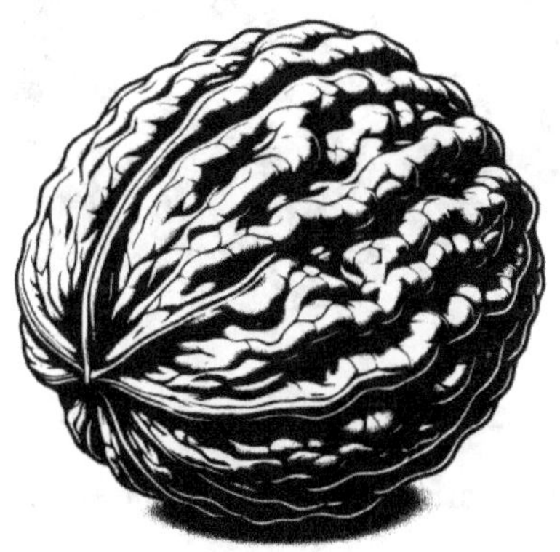

A dietary recommendation would be to consume 2-3 servings of raw or roasted nuts per day, with one serving equaling a handful (about 16 g). They can be consumed at any time of the day, though most people prefer to eat them during lunch or as a snack.

Remember that peanuts are not nuts but legumes. If consumed in large quantities, it's better to eat them roasted rather than raw, as like other legumes, they have antinutrients if consumed raw.

Fish

Consuming fish is related to a decrease in CVD risk. Specifically, it decreases the likelihood of having a sudden death episode in individuals with coronary heart disease. In addition to its omega-3 content, fish is also rich in vitamin D, selenium, and calcium. A good recommendation for the general population would be to consume 2 to 3 servings of fish per week. One serving of fish would be about 160 g net weight (a medium-sized salmon fillet, about 8 sardines).

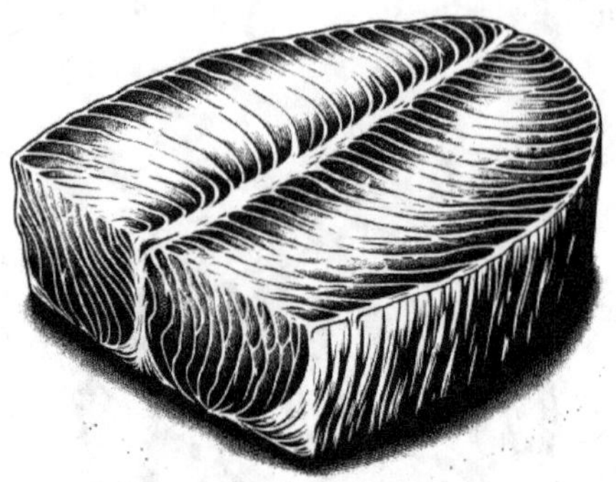

It is preferable to encourage the consumption of small-sized oily fish, such as sardines, anchovies, or boquerones. Salmon is also a good option. However, in the case of large-sized fish, attention should be paid to the possible contamination with methylmercury, especially if we are talking about swordfish, shark, red tuna or pike.

White fish such as cod, hake, monkfish, or sole are also good options, although their omega-3 content is lower than that of the small-sized oily fish mentioned above.

Whole Grains

Rice, oats, barley, rye, corn, spelt, and wheat are the most well-known grains in our environment. A whole or intact grain consists of three parts: outer covering or shell (bran), endosperm, and germ. Traditionally, the grains we consume in the form of pasta or bread are stripped of two of these parts, and we usually find them made only with the endosperm. The endosperm is rich in starch and has some protein. However, by removing the other two parts (bran and germ), we are reducing the nutritional quality of the grain since these fractions provide healthy lipids, vitamins, minerals, phytochemical compounds, and fiber.

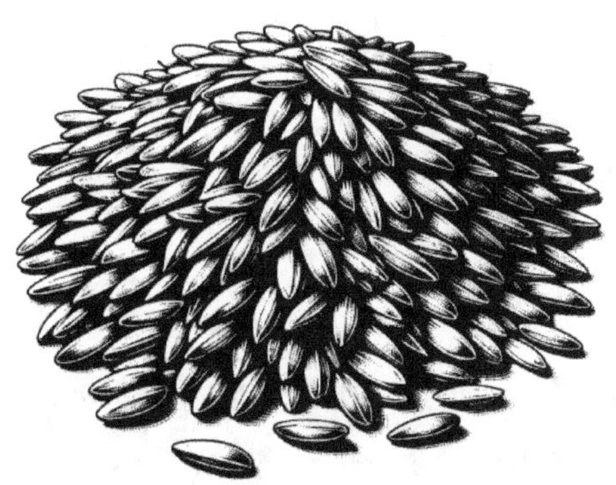

Similarly, consuming whole grain cereals is associated with a decrease in cardiovascular risk and overall mortality risk. Besides, consuming whole grains is related to:

- Better regulation of bowel movements.
- Benefits for our microbiota (also known as gut flora).
- Reduction and better control of blood glucose levels.
- Decreased risk of cancer (especially colorectal cancer).

Whole grains are not only good for "going to the bathroom," as many people think. If we started substituting the consumption of refined grains for whole grains, we would gain a lot in terms of health.

A relatively simple way to start incorporating whole-grain cereals into your diet is by buying whole-grain pasta instead of white pasta. The change in flavor is almost imperceptible as various types of side dishes and sauces usually accompany these dishes.

Finally, because "breakfast cereals" are often made with refined flour and lots of sugar, an option to replace them could be to consume whole grain cereal flakes, such as whole grain oats flakes.

Virgin Olive Oil

This oil should be the choice in all aspects of cooking, whether for dressing or frying. Its lipid profile and composition of antioxidant substances make it the preferred fat for these tasks, and for its healthy properties, it tolerates high temperatures well. Besides, extra virgin olive oil has been a staple of the Mediterranean diet for centuries. It has been shown in many studies to be a great ally for cardiovascular health.

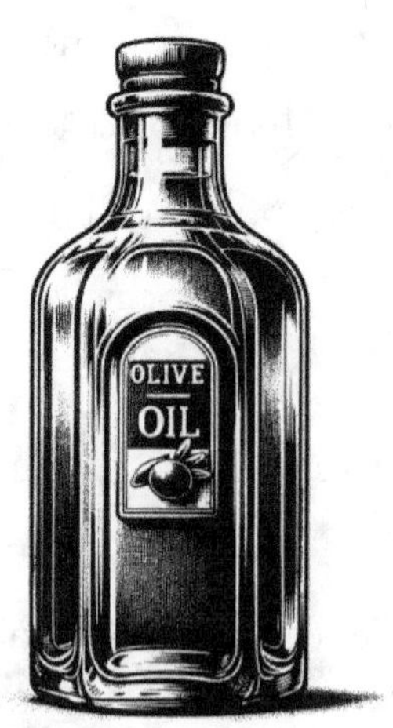

Fruits and Vegetables

Encouraging the consumption of fruits and vegetables is important because they provide fiber, antioxidant substances, vitamins, and various compounds associated with a decrease in overall mortality and cardiovascular risk. General recommendations could be to consume at least one serving of vegetables with each main meal (about two times a day, with one of these servings being raw vegetables) and at least 3 pieces of fruit a day.

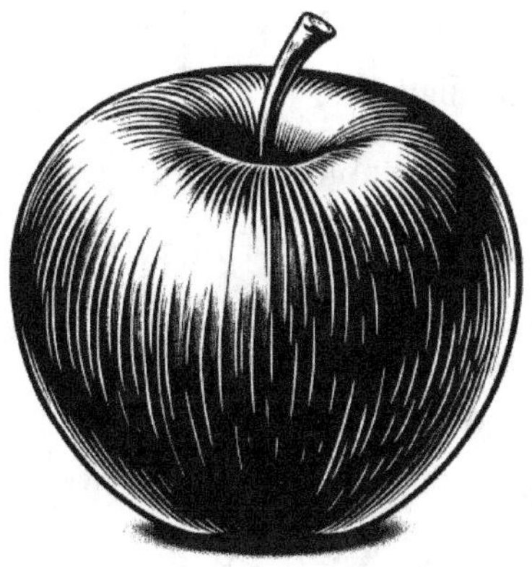

Fruits should be eaten whole and chewed, not only because chewing increases our feeling of fullness but also because consuming fruit in juice form leads to a more pronounced increase in blood glucose levels, followed by a spike in insulin. Consider this revealing example: normally, we cannot eat two large oranges. We might tire of chewing the segments before finishing the first one. However, it is much easier to drink juice made from 3 or 4 oranges at once. Even though the juice is made from the orange segments, retaining a lot of vitamins, the breakdown of the food matrix turns the sugar into free sugar, which does not trigger the same metabolic response as chewing the fruit. In summary, it's better to eat whole fruits than to drink them in juice form. Chewing fruits fills us up more (and is healthier) and doesn't raise our blood sugar as much as juice does.

Have you heard the myth, "Fruit contains sugars, so it's not recommended for people with diabetes"? As we've explained, fruits have sugars naturally present in them, with fructose being the most prominent. This has given rise to an unsupported myth. The American Diabetes Association (ADA) recommends a dietary pattern rich in fruits, vegetables, and whole grains (among others) for the proper management of diabetes.

So, considering the available scientific evidence, it doesn't seem logical to recommend excluding fruits from the diet of diabetes patients. But the recommendation of several pieces of fruit per day would be appropriate.

As for vegetables, their health benefits extend beyond their nutritional value. Studies have shown that a higher intake of vegetables, especially green, leafy, and non-starchy ones, can reduce the risk of chronic diseases such as certain types of cancer and heart disease.

Regular consumption of green leafy and cruciferous vegetables has been linked to a decreased risk of breast cancer. Additionally, incorporating a variety of vegetables in the diet may aid in the prevention and management of type 2 diabetes and contribute to gastrointestinal health. Some have also observed that vegetable consumption can positively influence weight loss and the maintenance of a healthy weight. Makes you want to eat them, doesn't it?

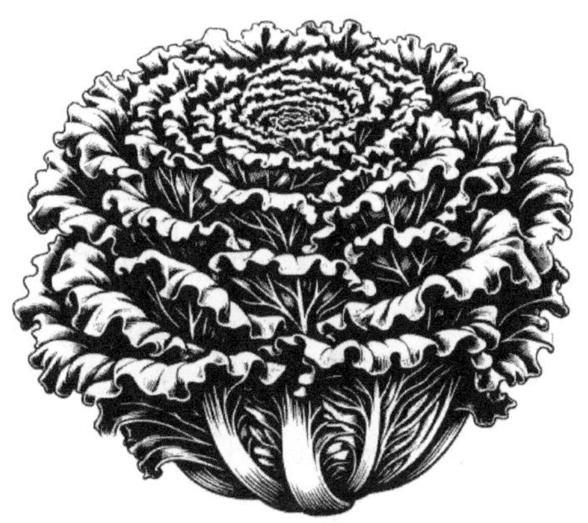

Another piece of advice would be to vary or combine fruits and vegetables based on their colors since this indirectly varies the content of different phytochemical compounds. The color of fruits and vegetables is usually a good indicator of their nutrient and phytochemical content. Each color in fruits and vegetables is associated with specific health benefits due to the unique compounds they have:

- <u>Red Fruits and Vegetables (like tomatoes, red peppers, strawberries, and apples)</u>: These are typically rich in antioxidants like lycopene and anthocyanins. Lycopene is known for its potential to reduce the risk of certain types of cancer, especially prostate cancer, and anthocyanins are beneficial for heart health.

- <u>Orange and Yellow Fruits and Vegetables (such as carrots, sweet potatoes, oranges, and bananas)</u>: These are high in vitamins C and A. Vitamin A is vital for eye health, and vitamin C is important for the immune system and skin health. They also have beta-carotene, which the body converts into vitamin A.

- <u>Green Vegetables (like spinach, kale, green beans, and broccoli)</u>: Rich in lutein, zeaxanthin, and vitamin K, these nutrients support vision health, promote strong bones, and may help lower the risk of certain cancers. Green leafy vegetables are also a great source of folate, which is essential for cell division and DNA synthesis.

- <u>Blue and Purple Fruits and Vegetables (such as blueberries, eggplants, and purple grapes)</u>: These foods are known for their high levels of antioxidants, particularly anthocyanins, which may help protect cells from damage and reduce the risk of heart disease, stroke, and cancer.

- <u>White and Brown Fruits and Vegetables (like cauliflower, garlic, and mushrooms)</u>: These often have phytochemicals like allicin (found in garlic), which have antiviral and antibacterial properties. They are also a source of potassium and dietary fiber.

I do not intend to overwhelm you with detailed information about micronutrients. The key takeaway I want you to remember is the importance of including fruits and vegetables in your diet and varying their colors. This simple approach, which I like to think of as 'eating the rainbow', is more than just a way to make your meals visually appealing; it's a practical strategy to ensure you're getting a diverse range of nutrients. So, if you can grasp this idea of embracing a colorful variety in your fruits and vegetables, I'll consider my job well done. This simple yet effective habit can make a significant difference in your overall health and well-being.

Legumes

Legumes such as chickpeas, lentils, beans, or soybeans are highly recommended foods due to their high content of protein, fiber, and plant sterols. Along with small fatty fish, they should be one of the main sources of quality protein for patients with high cardiovascular risk.

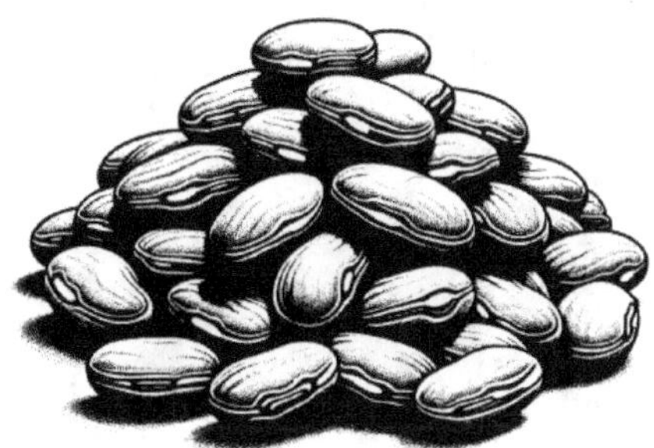

A serving of legumes would equal about 90 g raw and could be consumed at least 3 or 4 times a week. In case of difficulties cooking them, canned cooked legumes can always be used. After washing them well and removing excess salt, they can be consumed directly and are a quick and healthy option to accompany salads and other dishes or to prepare such as homemade hummus with chickpeas.

5

"NEUTRAL" FOODS FOR HEALTH

Eggs

The nutritional profile of eggs is interesting, not only due to their fatty acid composition, but also due to other aspects such as their high-quality protein and micronutrients. Additionally, as we have mentioned, dietary cholesterol (what we eat) has a relatively small impact on serum cholesterol levels (in our blood). This is reflected in the fact that, sometimes, up to one egg per day can be recommended. However, a sensible recommendation would be to consume a serving of eggs (one medium egg, about 60 g) 2 or 3 times a week to focus on the consumption of minimally processed plant-based foods. It should always be remembered that the rest of the diet should also be aimed at reducing cardiovascular risk. Obviously, eating scrambled eggs with vegetables is different from eating a cake that contains eggs (and refined flour, sugar, and low-quality fats), which highlights the importance of considering the broader nutritional context.

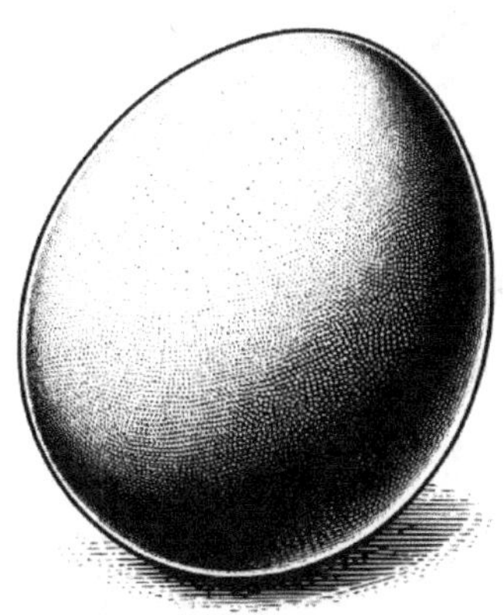

The vast majority of rigorous scientific studies agree that, at the population level, egg consumption is not associated with an increased risk of cardiovascular disease. It has been observed that up to seven eggs per week can be consumed with no problems by individuals without specific health issues. Additionally, incorporating eggs into the diet not only does not increase cardiovascular risk but could also function as a protective factor. This is generally due to their fatty acid composition, which makes the lipid profile of the egg nutritionally very compelling and minimally atherogenic.

Dairy Products

Consuming one serving of dairy per day (two yogurts or a glass of milk) is compatible with a diet to prevent cardiovascular risk. However, care should be taken with low-fat yogurts, as they often have added sugar or significant zero-calorie sweeteners.

So, it is preferable to consume whole, unsweetened yogurts (slightly protective in terms of cardiovascular risk). They can be accompanied by fruits, nuts, or whole grains. For example, a natural yogurt with strawberries, walnuts, and whole oat flakes is a great option for breakfast, dessert, or snack. As for milk, the main thing is that it is real milk, that is, pasteurized or UHT milk without added sugars. If you consume one glass of milk a day, whether it is skimmed, semi-skimmed, or whole, is unimportant, as the lipid profile of milk seems neutral. So attention should be focused on individual tastes and, above all, on what it will accompany the milk consumed.

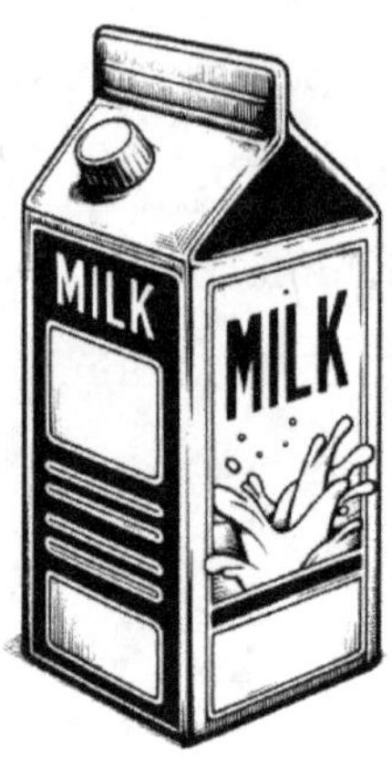

But if we talk about cheese, the recommendations would be different, not only because they are much richer in salt than yogurt or milk, but also because they have a higher fat concentration and are made with only a part of the protein fraction of milk, making them less nutritionally interesting. A serving of cheese is usually around two slices (60 g) as a garnish, and as a main dish, it usually equates to around four slices (120 g). About two servings of cheese per week could be consumed, focusing on low-salt and fresh cheeses over highly matured ones.

Coconut Oil

Coconut oil is a source of saturated fats, but as with dairy products, its medium-chain fatty acids have been shown to have health benefits such as increased metabolism and appetite reduction. In addition, coconut oil is resistant to high temperatures and can be used for high-heat cooking.

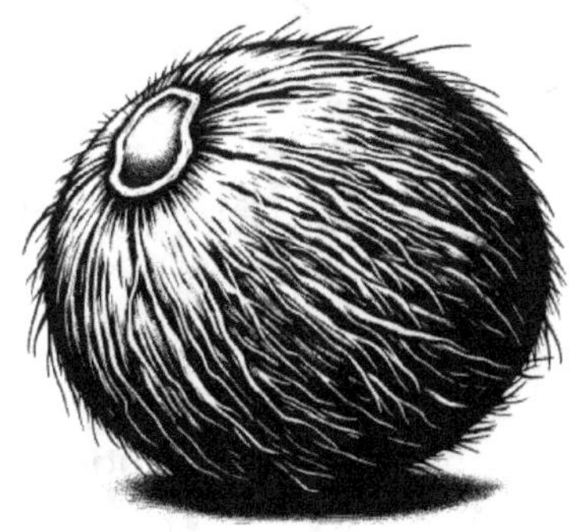

White Meat

Moderate consumption of white meat (rabbit meat and poultry such as chicken or turkey) is compatible with a healthy diet. A serving of about 120 g net weight (a medium-sized chicken breast fillet) can be consumed 2 to 3 times a week. However, it is advisable to go along with this meat with a serving of vegetables.

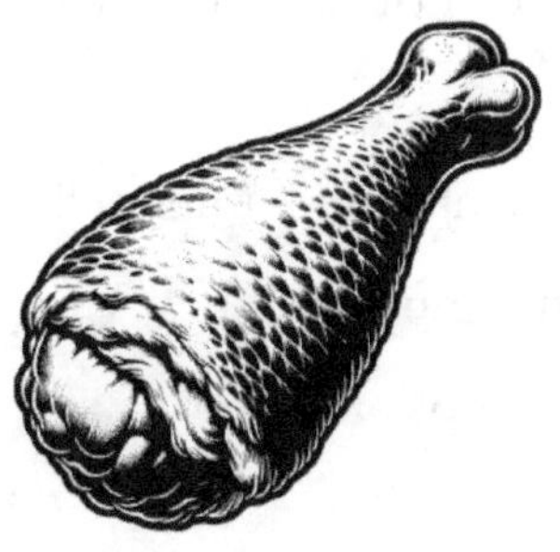

6

FOUNDATIONAL PRINCIPLES FOR A HEALTHY DIET

If we had to simplify the recommendations, we could base them on these premises:

- Avoid the consumption of ultra-processed foods, which are nothing more than ultra-palatable foods, usually made with refined flours, low-quality fats, salt, and sugar.
- Encourage the consumption of raw materials, that is, foods in a "similar" processed state to how we find them in nature. As comparative examples: a fillet of hake instead of breaded hake sticks, a steak instead of deli meat, whole fruit instead of juice, etc.
- Base the diet on plant-based, minimally processed foods (fruits, vegetables, legumes, nuts).
- Increase the consumption of foods rich in healthy fats, such as

extra virgin olive oil, avocado, nuts, and small oily fish.

- Consume whole grains and reduce the consumption of refined flours.
- Limit the intake of free sugars (table sugar, "soda" sugar, ultra-processed food sugar or juice).
- Although not dietary recommendations, because of their importance, it is worth mentioning that it is advisable to avoid tobacco and a sedentary lifestyle and engage in regular physical activity. A good sleep pattern and measures to combat stress would also be important.

What to change to eat healthier: 9 tips for a better diet

1

It's very useful to make a shopping list in advance following the guidelines, and once we're shopping, stick to the list. Similarly, if we go grocery shopping without hunger or having eaten something beforehand, we will avoid unhealthy temptations.

2

If we get used to shopping at the market instead of supermarkets, we will not only be buying local and seasonal products, but we will also avoid those shelves full of unnecessary products found in supermarkets.

3

When we buy non-raw food products, it is very important to check the ingredient list to make sure they do not contain added sugar, bad quality fats (palm, sunflower), refined flours, salt, etc.

4

When we buy nuts (raw or baked, not salted, fried or sugared) or dried fruit, we should check the ingredient list and make sure they comprise the raw material and little else.

5

A resource for having vegetables available every day could be to roast vegetables on a day when we have free time (like a Sunday, for example). We can make one or more trays, put the already roasted vegetables in containers and refrigerate them for when we need them.

6

In the same way as in the previous case, we can cut up several pieces of fruit in a day, put them in containers, and eat them later.

7

We can buy legumes either pre-cooked or not; both options are valid.

8

We can try different spices (nutmeg, garlic powder, onion powder, turmeric, parsley, rosemary) to decrease salt consumption.

9

It is essential not to have ultra-processed foods at home. If they are on hand, it is difficult not to resort to them if we have episodes of anxious hunger.

7

EFFECTIVE MEAL PLANNING FOR PROPER NUTRITION

Now we know which foods are healthy, which are not, and which we might consider neutral for health. We've also learned the basic principles of healthy eating. But now, a question may arise: how can we put all this into practice? Are there any useful tricks? Let's find out.

Simplification of Recipes

Start with simple dishes that require few ingredients. As you gain experience, you can explore more complex recipes. Begin with recipes that need less than five ingredients, preferably ones that can also be used in multiple dishes. For example, chicken, eggs, and certain vegetables are versatile and can be used in a variety of meals. One-pot or one-pan meals are excellent for beginners, as they simplify the cooking process and cleanup.

Let's see an example with a recipe for 'Grilled Chicken with

Vegetables and Whole Wheat Bread (for One).

<u>Ingredients:</u>

- 1 chicken breast (about 150-200 grams).

- 1-2 cups of your favorite vegetables (such as broccoli, carrots, bell peppers).

- 2 tablespoons of olive oil.

- Salt and pepper to taste.

- 1 slice of whole wheat bread.

<u>Instructions:</u>

1. <u>Prepare the Vegetables</u>: Wash and cut the vegetables into medium pieces. You can lightly steam them before grilling to soften them.

2. <u>Season the Chicken</u>: Season the chicken breast with pepper. You can add dried herbs like thyme or rosemary for more flavor.

3. <u>Cook the Chicken and Vegetables</u>: Heat a skillet over medium-high heat and add a tablespoon of olive oil. First, cook the chicken until it's golden and fully cooked, about 5-7 minutes per side. Then, remove the chicken and add the vegetables with more oil in the same skillet if needed. Cook until they are tender and slightly browned.

4. <u>Toast the Bread</u>: While the chicken and vegetables are cooking, you can toast the slice of whole wheat bread.

5. <u>Serve</u>: Place the chicken and vegetables on a plate. Accompany with the toasted slice of whole wheat bread.

This recipe is a perfect example of how a simple and healthy dish can also be delicious and satisfying. The key is in the quality of the ingredients and not overcomplicating the cooking process. This recipe is flexible, and you can adapt it based on the vegetables you have on hand or your preferences (you can do it, go for it!).

Storage and Organization

Investing in quality containers and organizing your food storage effectively can make meal preparation more efficient and enjoyable. Here are some tips and strategies to consider:

- Choose Quality Containers: Opt for airtight, high-quality containers. Glass containers are a great choice as they don't absorb odors and are easy to clean. They're also microwave and dishwasher-safe, making them convenient for various uses.

- Variety of Sizes: Keep an assortment of sizes for different needs. Smaller containers are perfect for sauces, dressings, or small portions of fruits and snacks. Larger containers are useful for complete meals, bulk ingredients, or family-sized portions.

- Labeling and Dating: Label your containers with preparation dates and contents. This helps you track when meals were prepared and reduce food waste. It's a simple yet effective way to keep your pantry and fridge organized.

- Fridge Organization: Place items that need to be consumed first at the front of your fridge. This ensures easy access and helps you remember to use items before they expire.

- <u>Using the Freezer</u>: Use your freezer to store meals for longer periods. This is especially helpful for batch cooking or when you have leftovers you won't be able to eat right away.

- <u>Meal Preparation According to Needs</u>: Prepare and store meals based on your weekly requirements. If you eat at home and with family most days, focus on storing larger portions. For individual meals, focus on single servings.

- <u>Regular Maintenance</u>: Regularly review and clean out your fridge and pantry. This helps in keeping your food storage spaces in order and making sure you're using items before they expire.

<u>Example: Preparing and Storing Chicken Vegetable Soup</u>

Imagine preparing a large batch of chicken vegetable soup. This nutritious option often tastes even better after a day or two. Use a large pot to combine chicken breast, low-sodium chicken broth, and a variety of fresh vegetables like carrots, celery, and spinach, along with herbs and spices. Once the soup is ready, divide it into individual portions. You can refrigerate some for the week and freeze the rest for future meals. This method saves time during the week and ensures you have healthy, ready-to-serve meals.

By following these tips, you'll find that managing your food storage becomes more streamlined, making your daily meal preparation smoother and more efficient.

Incorporating Variety in Ingredients

Incorporating a variety of ingredients into your meals is essential for balanced nutrition and enjoyable eating experiences:

- <u>Balance Nutrients and Flavors</u>: When planning your meals, strive to include a variety of foods that offer different nutrients and flavors. For example, pair quality protein like chicken, legumes, eggs, or fish with whole grains and a mix of vegetables.

- <u>Experiment with Colors and Textures</u>: Add color and texture to your dishes with fruits and vegetables of different hues. Each color not only makes the dish visually appealing but also contributes various vitamins and minerals, as discussed in previous chapters.

- <u>Include a Variety of Food Groups</u>: Ensure to include foods from all the main food groups: proteins, carbohydrates, and healthy fats (preferably less processed). This helps in creating balanced and nutritious meals.

- <u>Use Herbs and Spices</u>: Herbs and spices can add flavor and aroma without the need for excess salt or fats (and they're healthy!). Experiment with different combinations to find what you like best. Here are examples:
  - Basil: Ideal for Italian dishes, especially pasta and

pizzas. Pairs well with tomatoes and garlic.

o Oregano: Another Italian cuisine favorite. Great in sauces, roasts, and tomato-based dishes.

o Cilantro: Commonly used in Asian and Latin American cooking. Perfect for sauces, stews, and as a fresh garnish.

o Rosemary: Excellent for roasting, particularly with meats like lamb and chicken and potato dishes.

o Thyme: Versatile in soups, stews, and marinades. Works well with meats and vegetables.

o Parsley: Widely used in various cuisines. Great in soups, salads, and as a garnish.

o Turmeric: Known for its intense yellow color and used in curries and rice dishes.

o Black Pepper: A staple in any kitchen, ideal for most dishes.

o Cumin: Common in Mexican, Indian, and Middle Eastern cooking. Used in dishes like curries, chilis, and stews.

o Saffron: Highly valued for its unique color and flavor. Widely used in Spanish cooking, it's an essential spice in paella and other rice dishes.

o Cinnamon: Not just for desserts, also great in savory and spiced dishes.

o Ginger: Used in both sweet and savory dishes, particularly in Asian cuisine.

Imagine you're preparing a chicken and vegetable stir-fry. You can use chicken as your protein source, broccoli and red peppers for color and texture, and brown rice or quinoa as a carbohydrate base. For flavor, you might use garlic or ginger. This combination not only provides a variety of nutrients but also offers a rich and satisfying taste experience. But let's be even more practical. Here's a weekly food distribution with some example meals as a guide:

	FOOD	
BREAKFASTS	Coffee/tea/water/infusions Avocado/guacamole/hummus Grilled eggs Beans Oil Nuts Olives and pickles Cured cheeses Canned fish Whole milk and whole yogurts Hummus and nut creams Fruit	

LUNCHES	FOOD	EXAMPLES
Monday	Seafood	Grilled squid or shrimp with vegetables
Tuesday	White meat	Tomato salad and grilled chicken with spices
Wednesday	White fish	Pumpkin and carrot cream and baked sea bass
Thursday	White meat	Broccoli with Roquefort and stewed turkey
Friday	Bluefish	Sautéed spinach with garlic, onions, and salmon or tuna cubes
Saturday	Plant protein	Zucchini spaghetti with textured soy in Bolognese sauce
Sunday	Eggs	Zucchini and onion omelette

DINNERS	FOOD	EXAMPLES
Monday	Complete salad	Complete salad with goat cheese and walnuts
Tuesday	Bluefish	Baked salmon with vegetables
Wednesday	Eggs	Scrambled eggs with mushrooms and ham
Thursday	Seafood	White asparagus and boiled shrimp with chickpea hummus
Friday	Complete salad	Salad with tuna, lettuce, tomato, corn...
Saturday	Free	-
Sunday	White fish	Baked cod, hake or tilapia with a base of eggplants and baked spring onions

Optimizing Ingredients

Incorporating a variety of foods in your meal preparation can significantly enhance your dietary habits:

- <u>Cook a Variety of Foods at Once</u>: For example, when roasting vegetables, select a diverse range like zucchini, bell peppers, onions, broccoli, and carrots. Roasting them together provides a colorful and nutritious blend that can be used in multiple recipes.

- <u>Proper Storage</u>: Store your cooked items in airtight containers in the refrigerator or freezer, depending on your needs. This practice keeps them fresh and ready for use at any moment.

- <u>Creative Use</u>: Consider different ways to incorporate these foods. For example, roasted vegetables can serve as a side dish on their own, or you can add them to salads, pastas, stews, or as fillings for sandwiches.

<u>Practical Example with Roasted Vegetables</u>

Imagine you've roasted a large tray of assorted vegetables. Here's how you can use them throughout the week:

- <u>Monday</u>: Serve the roasted vegetables with some feta cheese and vinaigrette as a warm salad.
- <u>Wednesday</u>: Mix the vegetables with whole wheat pasta and your favorite sauce for a quick and healthy dinner.
- <u>Friday</u>: Use them as fillings for fajitas or tacos, adding beans and your choice of protein.

This approach is not just practical and time-saving, but it also ensures you consume a variety of vegetables throughout the week. Roasted vegetables can enhance the flavors of many dishes, making your meals more appetizing and varied. It's a win-win situation!

Plan Your Snacks

We all get hungry occasionally between the main meals of the day. Naturally, if we have unhealthy options at home, we're likely to choose these less desirable options (because they taste so good). The key lies in the grocery list. If it's not bought, it's not in the pantry, and if it's not in the pantry, it won't be eaten. Let's see then what we can buy as healthy snacks and some high-quality ideas and tips on how to integrate these snacks into your daily diet:

- <u>Fresh Fruits</u>: Fruits are an ideal snack because they are naturally sweet and full of vitamins, minerals, and fiber (and they're super healthy, as we've already seen). Examples include apples, pears, bananas, berries, and grapes. They are easy to carry and require no preparation.

- <u>Raw or Baked Nuts</u>: Nuts like almonds, walnuts, pistachios, and cashews are excellent sources of healthy fats, proteins, and fiber (and remember: they're not only healthy but also very filling and used in weight loss diets). Remember also: choose raw or oven-roasted versions without added salt to maximize nutritional benefits.

- <u>Vegetables with Hummus or Guacamole</u>: You can slice vegetables like carrots, cucumbers, and bell peppers and serve them with hummus or guacamole. This combination is not only tasty but also provides a good amount of fiber and healthy fats.

- <u>Edamame</u>: Edamame are immature soybeans and are a snack rich in protein and fiber. You can find them fresh or frozen, and they are easy to prepare.

- <u>Seeds</u>: Seeds, such as pumpkin or sunflower, are a nutritious snack that provides healthy fats, proteins, and minerals. Choose unsalted versions.

Being plant-based and minimally processed, these snacks contribute to a balanced and healthy diet. The key is variety and choosing options you like so you can enjoy these healthy snacks regularly.

Dedicate a Day for Planning and Shopping

Setting aside a specific day for meal planning and grocery shopping is an effective strategy that can make your weekly eating more manageable and healthier. Here's a detailed guide with practical tips:

- Choose the Day: Many experts recommend using the weekend for planning and shopping, such as planning on Friday, shopping on Saturday, and meal prep on Sunday. This approach helps organize the week without the pressure of work or school commitments.

- Menu Planning: Before going shopping, decide what meals you will prepare during the week. Consider your activities and commitments to choose recipes that fit your schedule and needs.

- Organizing the Shopping List: Organize your shopping list into sections according to the supermarket areas (e.g., fresh produce, pantry, meat/dairy, frozen). This helps you be more efficient and avoid forgetting items.

- Smart Shopping: Visit the inner aisles of the supermarket to find healthy options like legumes, vinegars, spices, olive oil, and frozen fruits and vegetables. Focus on fresh, unprocessed, or minimally processed foods, and pay attention to product labels. Be skeptical about claims like "low fat" or "reduced sugar". And one more thing: try to shop when you're not hungry! This way, you'll avoid being tempted by unhealthy choices.

- <u>Avoid Peak Hours</u>: Shopping during early morning hours on weekdays can result in a quicker and more relaxed experience, as stores are less crowded.

- <u>Flexibility in Plans</u>: Be flexible with your meal planning. While it's helpful to have a plan, you should also be willing to adapt, for example, if an ingredient isn't available or if there are changes in your schedule.

- <u>Incorporate Variety</u>: Try to include a variety of foods in your planning to ensure a broad range of nutrients and to keep your meals from becoming monotonous.

This guide offers a practical approach to weekly meal planning and grocery shopping, incorporating expert recommendations and practical insights. By following these steps, you can streamline your meal planning process, making it both efficient and enjoyable.

Strategies for Eating Out

Starting integrated strategies for eating out can help you enjoy your meals while sticking to healthy eating habits. Here's a detailed guide:

- <u>Review the Menu in Advance</u>: Before heading to the restaurant, check out the menu online and decide what you will order. Many restaurants and fast food chains now offer nutrition information on their websites, which can be a valuable tool in making healthy choices.

- <u>Choose Healthy Options</u>: Look for dishes labeled as healthy or light on the menu. Menus may have "healthy" designations or symbols or keywords in the names of some items (like light, fresh, fit, vegetarian, skinny) indicating healthier choices.

- <u>Ask About Dishes</u>: Don't hesitate to ask your server or even the chef about ingredients, preparation methods, or possible substitutions. Making healthy substitutions like using a red sauce instead of an Alfredo sauce in Italian dishes are easy ways to eat healthier while dining out.

- <u>Share or Take Home</u>: If portion sizes are large, consider sharing an entrée or setting aside half to take home before you start eating. This can help control portion sizes and prevent overeating.

- <u>Avoid Unnecessary Extras</u>: Resist the temptation of appetizers, cocktails, and complimentary bread and butter or chips and salsa, which can add extra fat, sodium, sugar, and calories.

- <u>Add Color and Nutrients</u>: Choose colorful fruits and vegetables as sides or substitutes for other ingredients in your dish. This not only makes the meal more visually appealing but also adds essential nutrients.

- <u>Ask for Healthy Oils and Dressings</u>: Ask about cooking oils used in the kitchen and ask for healthier non-tropical vegetable oils to be used instead. Also, ask for butter, cheese, toppings, salad dressings, sauces, and gravies to be served on the side so you control the amount used.

- <u>Nutritional Preferences</u>: Choose lean meats, whole-grain bread, and broth-based soups instead of heavier options. Select foods that are steamed, broiled, baked, roasted, poached, or lightly sautéed.

- <u>Maintain Healthy Habits</u>: Choose dishes like what you would eat at home and balance out other meals of the day if you plan to eat something heavier.

By following these guidelines, you can enjoy dining out without compromising your health and nutritional well-being. The key is planning, moderation, and making conscious choices based on your health goals and lifestyle. Remember, meal planning is an adaptable process and can be tailored according to your dietary preferences, cooking skills, schedules, and personal goals. With planning and preparation, you can ensure you're eating healthily and balanced, even on your busiest days, whether dining in or out.

8

ARE ADDITIVES HEALTHY?

If you've made it this far, it means you already have enough tools to make better decisions regarding grocery shopping. You now know that we should focus on raw materials, avoid ultra-processed foods and that an orange is healthier than juice. However, if you want to delve a little deeper into the world of nutrition, health, and the food industry, continue reading and learn a little more about the substances we will talk about now: additives.

What are Additives?

In its Codex Alimentarius, the Food and Agriculture Organization of the United Nations (FAO) defines a food additive as any substance that isn't typically eaten on its own or used as a main ingredient in food. These additives might not have nutritional value themselves, but when added to food at any stage - from production to storage - they might become a part of the food or affect its characteristics. This definition doesn't include contaminants or substances added to food for maintaining or improving its nutritional qualities.

However, the main reason the food industry uses additives is for technological purposes. These purposes can include:

- Extending the shelf life of foods, which means the food can be stored longer without spoiling.

- Altering the characteristics of food, such as its texture, color, or consistency.

- Enhancing the palatability or flavor, making the food taste better or different.

- Preserving the nutritional value, making sure the food keeps its vitamins and minerals during processing and storage.

- Additives are used to make food last longer, look and taste better, or to keep it nutritious. Authorities regulate these additives to ensure they are safe for consumption.

Are they safe?

As for the safety of consuming additives, it is worth mentioning something very relevant, which is that all additives present in foods marketed in both the United States and the European Union have undergone safety evaluations. In the European Union, these controls are carried out by the Scientific Committee on Food (SCF) and the European Food Safety Authority (EFSA).

But in the United States, the Food and Drug Administration

(FDA) is the government agency responsible for regulating and evaluating the safety of food additives. This agency establishes permitted limits of additives in food and conducts safety evaluations before approving them for use in food, as well as monitoring food additives once they have been approved to make sure they remain safe for food.

Before additives reach our supermarkets and restaurants, they have gone through control mechanisms that verify their safety and that they do not present risks to consumers at the doses at which they are usually consumed. In addition, the list of additives is sometimes re-evaluated to determine if there is new data on their safety, and in the event that any additive is found to cause any problem, it is withdrawn.

For the EFSA in Europe or the FDA in the United States to give the green light to use an additive and authorize it, it must be evaluated based on a dossier that must be submitted by the applicant for such authorization (for example, the company that wants to market the additive).

In addition, when the EFSA authorizes the use of an additive in Europe, it does so considering the maximum level intended to be used in different food products; in this way, using an additive can be restricted where the acceptable daily intake (ADI) is exceeded. Once the ADI of an additive has been identified and all tests to assess its safety have been passed, the European Union authorizes its use and categorizes it with an "E number", so that each specific additive will be easily identifiable in any member country. For example, vitamin C or ascorbic acid is E 300 in Europe, according to this classification.

In the United States, limits for food additives are set, and safety evaluations are conducted prior to their approval for food. Once approved, food additives are monitored to ensure they remain safe. Food additives are categorized as "generally recognized as safe" (GRAS) or approved food additives. GRAS additives are considered safe and do not require FDA approval before use, while approved food additives have gone through an approval process. Besides, approved food additives are identified by their chemical name, common name, or CAS number.

Using the same example as before, ascorbic acid (vitamin C) has the chemical name 2-oxo-L-threo-hexono-1,4-lactone-2,3-enediol, the common name "ascorbic acid," and the CAS number 50-81-7. It sounds very chemical, doesn't it? Well, it's nothing more than vitamin C we can find in oranges, mandarins, and strawberries, among others.

Therefore, that an additive corresponds to an "E number" or a CAS number does not mean it is artificial, much less so. Encompassing the set of additives, "E numbers," or CAS numbers within "chemical" or "synthetic" does not make sense, as this numbering is simply the result of a nomenclature aimed at standardizing food labeling. But something being artificial does not mean it is unhealthy, just as something natural is not automatically healthy. To combat chemophobia, many scientists have spoken out about it through books, campaigns, infographics, etc.

This is the case of Klaas Wynne, professor at the Faculty of Chemistry of the University of Glasgow, who created a graphic image showing an apple and, next to it, the list of "ingredients" it has completely naturally (with their respective "E numbers"). If we went to the field, saw an apple tree, picked any apple from it, and did a chemical analysis, it would have all these elements and compounds completely naturally. Logically, as we saw in the introductory chapter, an apple does not have a list of ingredients, since it is itself an ingredient or a raw material, just as an onion, a melon, celery, or a strawberry do not have a list of ingredients.

The goals for using food additives are primarily technological. The European Union legislation has classified these into 27 goals. Although, in a more summarized way, we could talk about colorings, preservatives, antioxidants, stabilizers, acidulants, flavor enhancers, and sweeteners.

Similarly, the FDA also categorizes food additives based on their function, which includes preservatives, colorings, flavorings, sweeteners, acidulants, emulsifiers, stabilizers, leavening agents, nutrients, and other additives. Each category refers to a specific objective that the food additive seeks to fulfill in the final product.

Colorants

Colorants are substances that give color to a food or restore its original color. Like other food additives, colorants can be "natural" or synthetic (the latter, being artificial, are usually more studied for greater safety in their use). Cochineal red (E 120), curcumin (E 100), or brilliant blue (E 133) are clear examples.

Some people with susceptibility may experience allergic reactions to the consumption of some colorants. Tartrazine or E 102 (lemon yellow color), for example, has been associated with allergenic effects, especially in asthmatic or urticarial people. Although it does not pose an excessive risk to the consumer from a toxicological viewpoint, some studies have linked it to negative effects on the activity and attention of children; for this reason, in Regulation (EU) No. 1333/2008 of December 16, 2008, it was decreed that labeling should have more information on this relationship when this colorant or others such as sunset yellow (E 110), quinoline yellow (E 104), carmoisine (E 122), allura red AC (E 129), and cochineal red A (E 124) were used in a food product. Years later (2013), a review entitled "Food additives and preschool children" was published in The Proceedings of the Nutrition Society, in which some stated that the relationship between the ingestion of these colorants and changes in children's behavior seemed evident if the observers were the parents. However, as for objective observers (who were not related to the children), there seemed to be no relationship (we can draw our own conclusions).

Another noteworthy case is the excessive and prolonged consumption of canthaxanthin (red colorant), which has been associated with retinal damage caused by the formation of crystals in the lipid membrane of the macula lutea. We would talk about very high doses, so nobody should be alarmed about this.

Preservatives

These extend the shelf life of food by protecting it from the attack and growth of microorganisms. An example would be lactic acid (E 270) or the curious case of boric acid (E 284), which was fraudulently used in the past to mask the darkening of shrimp and lobster heads.

This group also includes nitrates and nitrites, which are commonly found in processed meats. These compounds, if cooked at high temperatures and in the presence of amines, can transform into nitrosamines, which are not recommended due to their carcinogenic effect. So their amounts are specified and monitored in the final production phase of the food products in which they are used. Other controversial preservatives are sulfites, such as sodium sulfite (E 221). As for the use of sulfites as additives (present in processed meats, wines, some fruit juices, dried fruits, etc.), the EFSA has recommended further investigation, as the European population may be exceeding the ADI of these compounds (likely from consuming too many ultra-processed products). Excessive consumption of sulfites has been linked to hypersensitivity reactions, such as asthma, urticaria, or even angioedema. Again, we would be talking about very high doses of these compounds to produce these effects.

Antioxidants

Like preservatives, antioxidants also prolong the shelf life of food, but they protect against deterioration caused by oxidation (preventing color changes or rancidity in fats, for example). Antioxidants include ascorbic acid or E 300 (as we have seen, this is the famous vitamin C) and citric acid (E 330). Phosphates (such as phosphoric acid or E 338) are also included in this group, although they are also used as acidifiers and stabilizers. Excessive intake of phosphates can increase serum phosphorus (logically) and modify the phosphorus-calcium balance, so their consumption should be controlled in patients with chronic renal failure (CRF) or other important renal pathologies, where there should be exhaustive control of the intake of this mineral and many others.

Stabilizers

These are substances that preserve the physicochemical state of a food product. They are used to maintain a mixture between two immiscible substances or to keep the color of a food product, for example. Pectins (E 440) are stabilizers. Carrageenans (E 407), substances from algae that seem to be associated with worsening symptoms of inflammatory bowel diseases (IBD) such as Crohn's disease or ulcerative colitis, are also stabilizers. Studies in animals have indicated these compounds could cause typical histopathological alterations of IBD, modifying the intestinal microbiota, the intestinal epithelial barrier and stimulating the release of proinflammatory cytokines. Other studies carried out with human epithelial cells and microbiota seem to support the findings of the animal studies. Similarly, in a randomized clinical trial conducted between 2009 and

2013, published in 2017 in The Journal of Nutrition Health and Aging, it was found that the intake of carrageenans contributed to an earlier relapse in patients with ulcerative colitis in remission compared to patients who did not consume these substances. In conclusion, dietary restriction of carrageenans could help people with inflammatory bowel diseases. For the rest of the population, consuming these additives at the doses provided by legislation should not pose a greater problem.

Acidulants

They are used to give or increase the acidic flavor of a food product. Fatty acids (E 570) are an example. Some acidulants, such as sodium ferrocyanide (E 535), can be used only in salt and substitutes due to their toxicity. There are also acidity regulators, which regulate the acidity or alkalinity of food products.

Flavor enhancers

As the name suggests, these are used to enhance the taste and/or aroma of a food product. An example of a flavor enhancer would be monosodium glutamate (E 621), known for imparting umami flavor. This compound has been popularly associated with asthma, migraines, and "Chinese restaurant syndrome," but there is no scientific evidence to support these claims. Perhaps due to its addictive effect and its presence in ultra-processed products, the consumption of monosodium glutamate may be related to weight gain, as reflected in The China Health and Nutrition Survey.

Sweeteners

As almost everyone knows, they are substances used to give a sweet taste to foods or food products. They are also used as table sweeteners. They can be "natural" (such as thaumatin or E 957) or artificial (such as neotame or E961). Regarding their possible health effects, there seems ample scientific evidence linking some to alterations in energy balance and various metabolic functions. Similarly, they could affect oral and extraoral sweet taste receptors and alter various cognitive processes (reward mechanisms and perception of sweet taste). In addition, artificial sweeteners have been found to cause changes in the intestinal microbiota, promoting the proliferation of pathogenic microorganisms over non-pathogens. These changes in the microbiota are also related to different variations in glucose tolerance mechanisms. Scientific evidence suggests that there is an association between the risk of overweight or obesity and the consumption of artificial sweeteners. This connection has been identified through various studies, including meta-analyses. These facts seem to show that, to prevent and avoid overweight and obesity, we should avoid the use of artificial sweeteners (very present in light drinks, by the way) and increasingly get used to less sweet tastes.

Bibliography

Avasilcăi L, Cuciureanu R. Nitrates and nitrites in meat products-nitrosamines precursors. Rev Med Chir Soc Med Nat Iasi. 2011 Apr-Jun;115(2):606-11.

Azad MB, Abou-Setta AM, Chauhan BF, Rabbani R, Lys J, Copstein L, Mann A, Jeyaraman MM, Reid AE, Fiander M, MacKay DS, McGavock J, Wicklow B, Zarychanski R. Nonnutritive sweeteners and cardiometabolic health: a systematic review and meta-analysis of randomized controlled trials and prospective cohort studies. CMAJ. 2017 Jul 17;189(28):E929-E939. doi: 10.1503/cmaj.161390. PMID: 28716847; PMCID: PMC5515645.

Bhattacharyya S, Shumard T, Xie H, Dodda A, Varady K, Feferman L, et al. A randomized trial of the effects of the no-carrageenan diet on ulcerative colitis disease activity. Nutr Healthy Aging. March 31, 2017; 4(2):181-192.

Burke MV, Small DM. Physiological mechanisms by which non-nutritive sweeteners may impact body weight and metabolism. Physiol Behav. 2015 Dec 1;152(Pt B):381-388.

Cleveland Clinic. Your Guide to Healthy Meal Prep [Internet]. Cleveland: Cleveland Clinic; [cited 2023 Dec 14]. Available from: https://health.clevelandclinic.org/your-guide-to-healthy-meal-prep/

Dixit SG, Rani P, Anand A, Khatri K, Chauhan R, Bharihoke V. To study the effect of monosodium glutamate on histomorphometry of cortex of kidney in adult albino rats. Ren Fail. 2014 Mar;36(2):266-270.

EFSA.EU [Internet]. Parma: EFSA; 2011 [cited 2022 Apr 14]. Scientific Opinion on the substantiation of health claims related to olive oil and maintenance of normal blood LDL-cholesterol concentrations (ID 1316, 1332), maintenance of normal (fasting) blood concentrations of triglycerides (ID 1316, 1332), maintenance of normal blood HDL-cholesterol concentrations (ID 1316, 1332) and maintenance of normal blood glucose concentrations (ID 4244) pursuant to Article 13(1) of Regulation (EC) No 1924/2006. Available from: https://www.efsa.europa.eu/en/efsajournal/pub/2044.

EFSA.EU [Internet]. Parma: EFSA; 2016 [cited 2022 Apr 14]. Process contaminants in vegetable oils and foods. Available from: https://www.efsa.europa.eu/en/press/news/process-contaminants-vegetable-oils-and-foods.

EFSA.europa.eu [Internet]. Parma: EFSA; 2013 [cited 2020 Apr 10]. "Energy" drinks report. Available from: http://www.efsa.europa.eu/en/press/news/130306.

Elhkim MO, Héraud F, Bemrah N, Gauchard F, Lorino T, Lambré C, Frémy JM, Poul JM. New considerations regarding the risk assessment on Tartrazine An update toxicological assessment, intolerance reactions and maximum theoretical daily intake in France. Regul Toxicol Pharmacol. 2007 Apr;47(3):308-16. Epub 2007 Jan 10

European Parliament and Council of the European Union. Commission Delegated Regulation (EU) No 1169/2011 of 25 October 2011 on the provision of food information to consumers, amending Regulations (EC) No 1924/2006 and (EC) No 1925/2006 of the European Parliament and of the Council, and repealing Commission Directive 87/250/EEC, Council Directive 90/496/EEC, Commission Directive 1999/10/EC, Directive 2000/13/EC of the European Parliament and of the Council, Commission Directives 2002/67/EC and 2008/5/EC and Commission Regulation (EC) No 608/2004.

European Parliament and Council of the European Union. Commission Delegated Regulation (EU) No 1337/2013 of 13 December 2013 supplementing Regulation (EU) No 1169/2011 of the European Parliament and of the Council on the provision of food information to consumers as regards the indication of the country of origin or place of provenance of fresh, chilled and frozen meat of swine, sheep, goats and poultry.

European Parliament and Council of the European Union. Commission Delegated Regulation (EU) No 1333/2008 of 16 December 2008 on food additives.

European Parliament and Council of the European Union. Commission Delegated Regulation (EU) No 1129/2011 of 11 November 2011 amending Annex II to Regulation (EC) No 1333/2008 of the European Parliament and of the Council to establish a Union list of food additives.

European Parliament, Council of the European Union. Commission Delegated Regulation (EU) No 1169/2011 of 25 October 2011 on the provision of food information to consumers, amending Regulations (EC) No 1924/2006 and (EC) No 1925/2006 of the European Parliament and of the Council, and repealing

Commission Directive 87/250/EEC, Council Directive 90/496/EEC, Commission Directive 1999/10/EC, Directive 2000/13/EC of the European Parliament and of the Council, Commission Directives 2002/67/EC and 2008/5/EC and Commission Regulation (EC) No 608/2004.

FAO: Food and Agriculture Organization of the United Nations [Internet]. Definitions for the purposes of the Codex Alimentarius [updated June 10, 2017; cited June 11, 2017]. Available at: http://www.fao.org/docrep/w5975s/w5975s08.htm.

FESNAD-SEEDO. Evidence-based nutritional recommendations for the prevention and treatment of overweight and obesity in adults. 2012.

Foscolou A, Critselis E, Panagiotakos D. Olive oil consumption and human health: A narrative review. Maturitas. 2018; 118:60-66.

García-Villanova B, Guerra EJ. Cereals and derived products. In: Gil A. Nutritional Treatise. Volume II. Composition and Nutritional Quality of Foods. Madrid: Panamericana; 2005.

Harvard T.H. Chan School of Public Health. Meal Prep Guide [Internet]. Boston: Harvard T.H. Chan School of Public Health; [cited 2023 Dec 14]. Available from: https://www.hsph.harvard.edu/nutritionsource/meal-prep/

He K, Du S, Xun P, Sharma S, Wang H, Zhai F, et al. Consumption of monosodium glutamate in relation to incidence of overweight in Chinese adults: China Health and Nutrition Survey (CHNS). Am J Clin Nutr. June 2011; 93:1328-1336.

Ix JH, Anderson CA, Smits G, Persky MS, Block GA. Effect of

dietary phosphate intake on the circadian rhythm of serum phosphate concentrations in chronic kidney disease: a crossover study. Am J Clin Nutr November 2014 100: 1392-1397;2014.

Jakszyn P, Gonzalez CA. Nitrosamine and related food intake and gastric and oesophageal cancer risk: a systematic review of the epidemiological evidence. World J Gastroenterol. July 21, 2006;12(27):4296-303.

Jinap S, Hajeb P. Glutamate. Its applications in food and contribution to health. Appetite. 2010 Aug;55(1):1-10.

Mancini A, Imperlini E, Nigro E, Montagnese C, Daniele A, Orrù S, et al. Biological and Nutritional Properties of Palm Oil and Palmitic Acid: Effects on Health. Molecules. September 18, 2015;20(9):17339-61.

Martino JV, Van Limbergen J, Cahill LE. The Role of Carrageenan and Carboxymethylcellulose in the Development of Intestinal Inflammation. Front Pediatr. May 1, 2017;5:96.

Martyn DM, McNulty BA, Nugent AP, Gibney MJ. Food additives and preschool children. Proceedings of the Nutrition Society. Cambridge University Press; 2013;72(1):109–16.

Moore LW, Nolte JV, Gaber AO, Suki WN. Association of dietary phosphate and serum phosphorus concentration by levels of kidney function. Am J Clin Nutr. August 2015;102:444-453.

Quines CB, Rosa SG, Da Rocha JT, Gai BM, Bortolatto CF, Duarte MM, Nogueira CW. Monosodium glutamate, a food additive, induces depressive-like and anxiogenic-like behaviors in young rats. Life Sci. 2014 Jun 27;107(1-2):27-31.

Royal Decree 308/2019, of April 26, approving the quality standard for bread. Spanish Official State Gazette, No. 113, of May 11, 2019, pages 50168-50175.

Ruanpeng D, Thongprayoon C, Cheungpasitporn W, Harindhanavudhi T. Sugar and artificially sweetened beverages linked to obesity: a systematic review and meta-analysis. QJM. 2017;110(8):513-520.

Ruiz-Gutiérrez V, Morgado N, Prada JL, Pérez-Jiménez F, Muriana FJ. Composition of human VLDL triacylglycerols after ingestion of olive oil and high oleic sunflower oil. J Nutr. 1998 Mar;128(3):570-6.

Sanders T. Omega-6 Fatty Acids and Cardiovascular Disease. Circulation. 2018;139(21):2437-2439.

Schwingshackl L, Schwedhelm C, Hoffmann G, Lampousi AM, Knüppel S, Iqbal K et al. Food groups and risk of all-cause mortality: a systematic review and meta-analysis of prospective studies. Am J Clin Nutr. 2017 Jun;105(6):1462-1473. Available from: http://ajcn.nutrition.org/content/105/6/1462.long.

Shafaa MW, Diehl HA, Socaciu C. The solubilisation pattern of lutein, zeaxanthin, canthaxanthin and beta-carotene differ characteristically in liposomes, liver microsomes and retinal epithelial cells. Biophys Chem. 2007 Sep;129(2-3):111-9.

Song P, Wu L, Guan W. Dietary Nitrates, Nitrites, and Nitrosamines Intake and the Risk of Gastric Cancer: A Meta-Analysis. Nutrients. 2015 Dec 1;7(12):9872-95.

Suez J, Korem T, Zeevi D, Zilberman-Schapira G, Thaiss CA,

Maza O et al. Artificial sweeteners induce glucose intolerance by altering the gut microbiota. Nature. 2014 Oct 9;514(7521):181-6.

Suez J, Korem T, Zilberman-Schapira G, Segal E, Elinav E. Non-caloric artificial sweeteners and the microbiome: findings and challenges. Gut Microbes. 2015;6(2):149-55.

Sujak A. Exceptional molecular organization of canthaxanthin in lipid membranes. Acta Biochim Pol. 2012;59(1):31-3.

Pearlman M, Obert J, Casey L. The Association Between Artificial Sweeteners and Obesity. Curr Gastroenterol Rep. 2017 Nov 21;19(12):64. doi: 10.1007/s11894-017-0602-9. PMID: 29159583.

Vojdani A, Vojdani C. Immune reactivity to food coloring. Altern Ther Health Med. 2015;21(Suppl 1):52-62.

World Health Organization. Guideline: Sugars intake for adults and children. WHO; 2015.

Wu JHY, Marklund M, Imamura F, Tintle N, Ardisson AV, De Goede J, et al. Omega-6 fatty acid biomarkers and incident type 2 diabetes: pooled analysis of individual-level data for 39,740 adults from 20 prospective cohort studies. Lancet Diabetes Endocrinol. December 2017;5(12):965-974.

About the Author

Glenda K. Ashworth is a nurse and dietitian driven by a profound commitment to health, education, and inspiring positive change. With her extensive background in medical care and nutritional science, Glenda has dedicated her career to empowering individuals to take control of their health through informed dietary choices.

A fervent advocate for heart health and balanced nutrition, Glenda's approach in "Easy Eating" combines her clinical expertise with a deep understanding of the everyday challenges people face in maintaining a healthy diet. Her work reflects a unique blend of scientific rigor and practical wisdom, making the complex world of nutrition accessible to all.

In "Easy Eating," Glenda not only shares her knowledge but also her personal and professional experiences, providing readers with a relatable and trustworthy guide. Her writing embodies a compassionate understanding of the diverse dietary needs and preferences that make each person's journey to health unique.